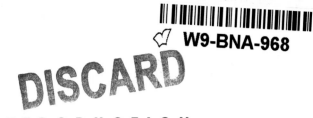

INTRODUCTION

SHOW ME WHERE BEAUTY IS

Women of African descent live with a bizarre duality when it comes to the beauty ideal. Folks say that the qualifications for "Beauty" in the dominant culture have opened up. You can now be a brunette and be considered beautiful! You've come a lo-ong way, baby! Folks also tell us that beauty standards in the black culture have opened up as well. First it was light skin with white features and naturally straight hair. Then it was Black Is Beautiful, which for many of us was rather short-lived.

Then the color qualification gradually broadened to include darker shades, but the features still had to be Caucasian. This is what is being termed an "*un*conventional, conventional" beauty, I guess, because it is "unconventional" to consider extremely dark skin "beautiful."

Black women with big lips or wide noses are considered to have an "ethnic" beauty. White women with big lips and noses have a "quirky, offbeat" beauty. This is about novelty and hype because the "quirky ethnics" are still being measured against the same old baseline.

It is not only the dominant culture that is guilty of perpetrating a narrow and frustrating beauty standard; black people contribute a fair share of support and reinforcement as well. I've been in movie theaters and actually heard not only the young black men but the black *women* comment—and I must say, rather loudly—on how "ugly" a dark-skinned actress is on the screen. And these are not actresses made up to play "ugly" roles, either. The actresses they refer to are usually dark skinned with African features and/or unprocessed hair. I have always made an effort to get a look at some of these commentators and have seen that quite often they themselves shared the same features as the actress they were ridiculing.

So what's new? I'm tired of hearing about how "unfair" everything is and how "we should all be accepting" and "we are all beautiful." I realize that you can't have a notion of physical "beauty" without some kind of standard defining what "beauty" is; that's just the way it goes. We know that it will be a long time, if ever, before we see an ebony-skinned, clearly Rubenesque, short-'froed woman with big lips and an African nose strutting down the runway wearing the crown and carrying an armful of roses at the Miss America pageant. If white women who weigh more than a hundred and five pounds are shut out of the mix, you can best believe it isn't going to happen for us. And that's okay; every culture has its fantasy ideal, and this is the stuff that legends are made of.

Even though demeaning standards exist in the black community, there have always been plenty of women who have flourished in spite of them. You can probably even think of women you've heard of or know of who don't fit the so-called ideal but have gotten over big time because they refused to swallow the beauty party line. The ones with the dark skin *and* the wide noses. The tall and thin ones with small breasts and skinny legs. The ones with the nappy short hair. The ones with large behinds and breasts—an exaggerated hourglass shape. Other black women would talk about them, saying:

> "I don't know *what* he sees in that *black, nappy-headed thing!*"
> "She is entirely *too big* to be wearing *that!*"
> "She *needs* to cover up those *bird legs.*"

And before they knew it, they'd be looking at Bird Legs in a magazine layout, their man had left them to be with Too Big, and Nappy had gotten the job that they'd bought that hairweave to get. This was even more of an outrage to women whose own lack of imagination and fortitude had left them choking in the dust. They just couldn't figure it out—*those* women didn't *deserve* to be admired; *we* knuckled under and used the bleaching cream, so why should *they* be rewarded? Could it be because they weren't sitting around, waiting for approval? It's time to stop complaining and wishing. The rules have changed but the game has stayed the same. So make up a game that you can play.

There are a lot more choices for black women now. Sometimes it takes strength and character to make those choices, but they do exist. Back in the day, everyone had a degree in kitchen cosmetology because we had *no choice;* not only were you expected to measure up to the Impossible Dream, you had to mix up your own products to make it happen because the mainstream cosmetics companies weren't interested in your business. You had to wear somebody's ashy-red Suntan or you learned how to mix different shades from different cosmetics lines or you didn't wear foundation. Unstraightened, tightly coiled hair was considered unfeminine, radical, militant, offensive, and ugly. If your hair burned off from hot-combing or broke off from a chemical straightener, you *had no choice:* You wore a wig or you were subjected to public ridicule.

Today you can be kitchen beautician by choice; it's because you like making your oatmeal cleanser and because you know that an olive oil treatment is good for your hair. If you don't like straightening your hair, you can get braids, wear the short-cropped natural, grow some locks, or twist up some coils. You can get some foundation from Fashion Fair, Naomi Sims, Flori Roberts, or Iman. And if they don't have what you want, you can have your own custom-blended at the Prescriptives counter. You don't have to look two shades lighter or wear sky-blue eye shadow now because *you have a choice.*

The French have an old phrase that refers to a woman who doesn't fit the standard of conventional beauty but whose allure and desirability factor turns heads no matter what her age. It is *jolie laide,* which means "beautiful-ugly," and can be used to describe an otherwise plain woman who has taken whatever it is about her that makes her "ugly" and turned it into an asset that allows her to compete with the blondest of the blondes. I am not saying here that black women are ugly; I am saying that since being black in and of itself shuts a lot of us out, the healthiest thing to do is to keep your head up and move forward. This *jolie laide* attitude not only works for women who are considered plain but can be useful for women who feel they are hopelessly out of the running even though they *are* attractive or they *are* pretty but are constantly being fed the message that the beauty of the dominant culture is "better."

The woman who doesn't fit the beauty ideal doesn't waste her time and spirit feeling unworthy. Her skin may be flawless, so she plays that up. Her legs and feet may be pretty, so she wears exquisite shoes and sheer hose and skirts a little above the knee. Her thin body and flat chest allows her to wear a sleek dress with a plunging back. A short, plump, big-chested woman watches her diet so things don't get completely out of hand, but she plays up those curves instead of collecting a wardrobe of muumuus. Her big lips are outlined and tantalizingly colored. Her plump, high, jutting behind is encased in well-fitting jeans. Her ebony skin gleams because she polishes it with stimulating salt scrubs, soaks in a milk bath, and pampers it with moisturizers. Her chronically damaged hair has been shaped into a chic cropped cut. Or the short, nappy hair that "refused" to grow into the shoulder-length straightened bob now flows past the shoulders in beautifully coiled locks. And she develops her mind and her wits so she has even more to offer.

I, along with many other black women, have struggled through the self-image and beauty maze. I have stumbled from time to time and will probably do so again, and yet I try to remember to keep my head up and look for inspiration wherever I can find it. But you must keep this in perspective: If you allow the world to tell you that you must fit into an uncompromising ideal, then you're going to become lost and bitter. You're the one who should show yourself where your own beauty is, and then everyone else will fall into line behind you.

The
Kitchen
Beautician

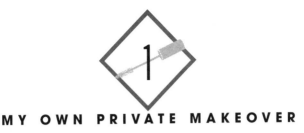

MY OWN PRIVATE MAKEOVER

Black women have had a history of creating beauty products for themselves when none existed. We are used to darkening that bottle of Suntan foundation, browning up that pot of cherry-red rouge. There are more choices in today's world, but fitting into the mainstream ideal is still a game of "touch and go." I found it doubly hard growing up, because although I lived in integrated neighborhoods and attended integrated schools, black wasn't beautiful unless you were "a Diana Ross." My beauty agenda was off course until Cleopatra Jones and Coffy came along and I got an Afro wig and a fake-fur battle jacket.

I needed a makeover that went beyond applying an egg-white mask and propping my elbows in lemon cups. I had a profound dissatisfaction with the way I looked. I wanted "beauty," and from all visible indications I had fallen short in every category. My large forehead and slightly bulging eyes earned me the hated nickname of Tweety. My adolescent features were morphing from week to week, but the only constant I could see was my nose, which was way too big and too flat. I saw my body as thin and shapeless, with no evidence of the rounded butt or big legs that were considered attractive and alluring, and I didn't think my breasts would ever make an appearance. Some wag noted that I "didn't have enough behind to make a good-sized hamburger." Having guys call me Miss Highpockets did not have the same flavor as shouting out "Baby's got back!" And the hair? I actually wrote a book about it: *Good Hair: For Colored Girls Who've Considered Weaves When the Chemicals Became Too Ruff.*

Whenever I tried to re-create any of those magazine "makeover secrets," I stumbled and fell, again and again. Much of my failure had to do with having an extremely limited budget, unrealistic expectations, and a refusal to embrace my physical attributes. I was determined to create the *new beautiful me* that would, first, humble my parents into renouncing their membership in the "I Said No" club and, later, forever ensure my popularity and attraction to the opposite sex. There was only so much that Fashion Fair, Posner, and Flori Roberts could do; my mission was to undertake a series of self-improvement projects of my own.

The Hairline Makeover

There were days when I simply couldn't get my hair together, days when all I could do was pull it back into a reasonable facsimile of a bun. I could cheat a bun by stuffing a crocheted bun cover with dark tissue paper, but my hairline was out in the great wide open for all to see. A severe case of Chemical Relaxer Revenge had caused my hairline to recede farther back than George Washington's. Long before spray-on hair was available, people—okay, vain older men—would darken their mustaches and graying, thinning hair with shoe polish.

The Hair Makeover Hall of Fame—This special mention goes to Yvonne Rhetta. Yvonne deserves a special mention because of the determination and sheer willpower she demonstrated in her early quest for "beauty." Yvonne tells her story:

"Y'know, back in the day, your hair had to be so pressed, so straight. I remember I'd wear my hair up in a big ponytail, but your kitchen would nap up when you'd wash your neck. I wasn't allowed to press my own hair between visits to the beautician, but I had this nappy kitchen, so I took a razor and shaved my neckline, except I ended up shaving *way* up my neck! I had shaved pretty far up, so I couldn't hide it, I just had to wait for my hairline to grow back. I got into a *lot* of trouble for that."

I was desperate, but visions of Al Jolson crept into my mind at the thought of shoe polish, and if it was discovered, I'd never live it down. I went for the next best thing, the cheapest wand mascara that money could buy. It was a perfect deception; the mascara wand would mimic strokes of the desperately needed hair on my hairline and in the process thicken the existing hairs, since that's what it was designed for anyway.

But nonwaterproof mascara is not designed to stand up to strong sunlight and sweat. I was at a noontime concert when a friend asked me if I'd recently dyed my hair. I ran to the bathroom and saw brown rivulets sliding down my temples. I wiped away half my foundation trying to clean up the mess, and my carefully plastered-down

---

The Hair Makeover Hall of Fame—This special mention goes to Martha R. Blanding, whose inventiveness in the face of cattiness goes unchallenged. Consider the fact that she pulled this off in the Dark Ages, before hairweaves and extensions became commonplace. I'll let Martha tell her story.

"Remember curlicues? The style where you pulled your hair back in a bun and had little ringlets above the ears and your forehead? Well, I had plenty for the bun, but I didn't have any hair for the edges, so I used to make curlicues. I used to clip pieces of hair out of one of my mother's wigs and curl them in a curler. Then I'd take eyelash glue and glue the curled ringlets along my hairline. I'd fix my hair around the edges so you couldn't see the glue, and they looked really natural. The eyelash glue would just peel away, so they were easy to get out. Only my close buddies knew I was doing it, and I worked my curlicues for a long time." But then the truth came out.

"I was on the dance floor at a party and one of my curlicues fell out in front of everybody. They all laughed, but it was okay. I just picked it up and kept on partying."

hairline sprang up into attention. I cadged a dab of Vaseline from a sympathetic girl in the bathroom and smoothed everything down the best I could, which had the effect of highlighting every thinning, shining patch of missing hairline. And there I was—exposed, with no scarf, hat, or anything. I thought quickly—sunglasses! Thank goodness for coolness! I perched my sunglasses on top of my head, Jackie O style, and slipped out of the bathroom. I went back to class and for the rest of the day I pretended I'd forgotten that my glasses were on top of my head.

The Body Makeover

Today the focus is on weight loss, but when I was growing up, the problem was getting a shape, some dangerous curves. In black culture, being bone-thin is not considered a great asset. I was straight up and down, and when the Flatsie doll came out—Flatsie looked like a pale Gumby with long hair—she became the bane of my existence. "Flatsie, Flatsie, she's flat, and that's that!" If I couldn't have breasts just yet, maybe I could do something about my shape. First off, I noticed that the models were skinny but had curves where their waists and hips were. Then I noticed that their navels didn't poke out; they had "innies." I had a protruding "outie," which caused me great anxiety when it came time for midriff tops and two-piece bathing suits. I asked around and my friend Vickie's mother told me that when a baby's navel wouldn't turn in, you'd tape a nickel down on top of it and the pressure would make it go in. If a nickel worked for babies, then I figured that a quarter would work for me. I taped a quarter to my outie with some surgical adhesive tape, shaped in an ✕, and was careful to keep it covered day and night for about three weeks. I checked it every night to see how it was coming along. Now it was time to put phase two of my makeover into action—the shape problem. I began doing waist stretches and pulls to encourage some kind of waist indentation.

One day, I lifted my arms to reach for something and my mother saw the big surgically taped ✕. What on earth had happened to me? What had I gone and done? "Mom, it's only a quarter. I'm wearing a quarter on my navel."

And just exactly what did I think this would accomplish?

"I'm turning my navel in," I said matter-of-factly. "You know, like they do for babies. So it'll be an *innie*."

My mother nodded slowly and turned around rather quickly, saying she had to "check on something." She didn't get away fast enough, though—I could see her shoulders shaking with laughter. Well, she'd see who laughed last when I showed her my new innie. I wore my quarter for weeks, until she finally broke it down to me that the coin bit worked for newborns—sometimes—because their navels were still umbilical stubs, but once that healed, you were stuck with whatever you ended up with. It wasn't until I started checking out the models in *Essence* magazine that I realized she was right, and girls with outies were wearing their midriffs and bikinis with the best of the innies. But I kept on with the daily waist stretches; no one had to know about that.

The Nose Makeover

In my preteen years, my features changed from week to week, but the one constant was my nose. It fits my face now, but then all I saw was my wide Brittenum nose. I had heard of Jewish and Italian girls getting nose jobs, but to actually say that you wanted a different nose was considered politically incorrect in the black community. Even though attitudes have changed somewhat, there is still a lot of debate on the subject. To me, this was a case of wanting something but being afraid of public opinion, and that feeling wasn't exclusive to blacks. Caucasian girls who showed up at school in bandages were fond of claiming that some tragic blow to the nose had necessitated a cosmetic rhinoplasty. I only knew of a few girls who just said it plain and declared that they had had the surgery because they'd agonized over their noses and they wanted the improvement. No problem, no guilt trip.

Somewhere, about the same time I started the navel makeover, I was eavesdropping and heard my mother say that in the olden days, when a baby's nose was wide, mothers would put the unhinged end of a clothespin on the bridge of the nose to narrow it down. This supposedly worked because of the malleable condition of the baby's nasal cartilage. I interpreted that to mean that I'd better get started now, while my cartilage was still young. Muhammad Ali could land a roundhouse dead on my nose and my parents—whose motto was "Money doesn't grow on trees"—*still* wouldn't shell out for a nose job. ("You'd better *wear* this clothespin and be quiet!") If my mother had taken care of business when I was in diapers, I wouldn't have this problem. First she lagged on my navel and now this.

Because time was a-wasting, I began wearing my clothespin around the house and sleeping with my mouth open at night. Sometimes I'd wake up with the impression of a clothespin on my cheek, because it had popped off my nose while I was sleeping. That was a problem that had to be taken care of immediately because those eight hours of continuous pressure were key in making my low-budget rhinoplasty work. So I anchored my clothespin with two strips of surgical tape and slept on my back. This wasn't always successful, and sometimes I'd have pieces of tape stuck to my face along with the clothespin imprint, but it worked most of the time.

I could only wear my clothespin sporadically during daylight hours because (1) I didn't want to be busted by my friends and (2) I didn't want my mother to stop me from wearing it. The friends situation? No problem. I always removed it before going out. The mother situation was more of a challenge. I had been wearing the clothespin in the confines of my room for about a week, removing it to run to the kitchen or bathroom, so it was like my mother saw it but really didn't see it. I kind of assumed that because she knew about the idea, she'd naturally approve. But she surprised me. Once she actually saw what I was doing, she didn't give me a hard time about it. I guess by that time she figured I'd eventually tire of it and move on to something else. And as soon as I removed the last of the tape residue and grew tired of giving my nose sponge baths to remove the marks left by the clothespin, I gave it up. But I hadn't heard the last of it. One day my mother was conversing with the mother of a friend whose nose was more in line with what I thought mine should have been.

"You know, Lonnice was wearing a clothespin on her nose. Now

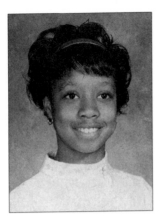

The bane of my adolescence, the Brittenum nose.

she says she wants one of those nose jobs! She doesn't need that!" clucked my mother as the girlfriend's mom shook her head in sympathy.

I could have died of embarrassment. My girlfriend Tina (a pseudonym) already *had* a perfect nose! Why did my mother have to say that? Just as I began to sink under a chair, I heard something that made me bob back up again.

"Really? Well, Tina has been asking for one, too. What do you think of that?"

The Wardrobe Makeover

Since I was on a tight budget while growing up, I tried to stretch my wardrobe by sewing. I had girlfriends who sewed quite well and turned out some fashionable outfits, often out of remnants. One could scare up a few dollars for fabric and a pattern, but you had to have a sewing machine; the days of sewing entire garments by hand were over. The girls I knew who sewed had access to their mothers' machines or owned one of their own. My mother had a sewing machine, but I wasn't allowed to use it. She did, however, present me with the latest model that Ronco had to offer. Those who are familiar with the Veg-O-Matic and the Buttoneer will quickly recall another Ronco offering, a hand-held, battery-operated sewing machine. The ads pointed out that Ronco's lightweight, plastic, portable sewing machine could perform tasks that the standard machine couldn't. Has that lace edging on your tablecloth fallen off minutes before your dinner party? Whip out the Ronco and you can stitch it back right there at the table with the first course steaming on top of it! Has the hem fallen out of your skirt minutes before the party guests are due to arrive? Dry those tears and whip out your Ronco—it's so easy, your husband can hem your skirt and you don't even have to take it off! The spiel focused on piecework; I didn't notice an emphasis on creating an entire garment, although the Ronco ads implied that it was certainly possible to do so. For $14.95 (or something like that) my parents were willing to give it a try.

The ads proclaimed that you never had to deal with "those pesky bobbins." That's because the only stitch possible on a Ronco was a primitive chain stitch. Instead of the understitched seam, which shows a running stitch on both sides of the seam, the underside of a chain-stitch seam shows interlocking loops or chains of thread. If you pull the end thread, all the loops come out and the entire seam unravels. The last stitch must be "locked"; this means a sewing needle is used to pull the end thread through the last loop on the underside of the seam. Every seam had to be locked, which made sewing anything other than an occasional tablecloth hem a tedious business. Without that "pesky bobbin," the Ronco turned out to be one step above hand sewing. But I had asked for a sewing machine, and technically I had received one. It was time to get busy.

I was meeting friends at the pizza joint and the rage was drawstring pants. I had my Simplicity pattern and my remnant. I ran up the pants on my Ronco. I carefully locked each seam and double-stitched the inseam. The pants fit and for once I had something stylish that I hadn't had to hound my parents into buying. Besides, the gathered, drawstring waistband gave the illusion of my having a behind that was a Burger King Whopper instead of a White Castle hamburger. It was the beginning of a whole new era.

"Yeah, girl, I just ran these up on the machine. They finally gave me one."

I was having a good time at the pizza joint and it was a breezy late-summer evening, so it was quite a while before I noticed the air on my upper thighs. I looked down in my lap and saw that the breeze had apparently blown right through the inseam of my pants. I excused myself and headed for the bathroom. The flimsy chain stitch gave way with every step I took, and by the time I made it to sanctuary, my entire inseam was gone. The only parts that remained intact were the drawstring waistband and the side seams. I ran into a stall, pants flapping open like a pair of crotchless chaps, my bare legs and panties completely exposed. The double-stitched, locked seams had disintegrated and two extremely long threads were all that were left. I grabbed them.

Poking my head out of the bathroom, I called a girlfriend over, and once she was in loud whispering range, told her that I'd split my pants a little bit. Could she get me a needle or something? She returned with Scotch tape and paper clips, which I grabbed from her, then slammed back into the stall. It was either do, or die of humiliation if I couldn't. I wasn't about to tell anyone that the pants I'd made with a Ronco sewing machine had fallen apart. I couldn't even cover my butt with a jacket because I didn't have one. The tape wasn't enough to hold the inseam on its own. What could I do with paper clips and the hanging inseam threads? Cursing Ronco and Mr. and Mrs. Bargainmeister, I removed my pants and sat down on the toilet seat. I straightened out a paper clip and wound an inseam thread around the base of it, as if it were a big needle. Holding the fabric edges together, I poked the paper clip through the fabric and dragged the thread through to the other side. The effect was a very crude Flintstones whipstitch, secured by a lot of thigh-scratching Scotch tape. It wasn't couture, but it got me through the evening without total embarassment.

When I got home and told my mother about the fiasco, she said I should have double-stitched and locked the seams.

"You have to take the *time* to do the job *right* when you sew, Lonnice."

I let the batteries swell and rust inside the Ronco, making sure that they were leaking pretty good before ditching it, lest my parents object to me throwing away a "perfectly good machine" and

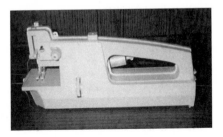

Believe it or not, my parents bought another Ronco sewing machine.

insisting that I use it. A year later, I received a real sewing machine, which I took with me when I went away to college. I continued my wardrobe makeover and, in retrospect, realize I turned out some pretty tacky stuff, but none of it fell apart.

COMFORTABLE IN YOUR SKIN

The greatest beauty asset that we have been blessed with is our skin. The extensive palette of Negroid skin has a built-in beauty enhancement called melanin. Some people have assigned a spiritual value to melanin and there's nothing wrong with that, I suppose, but melanin has a perfectly respectable physiological explanation as well. It doesn't hurt to become informed about it. In fact, it can only help you maintain your good looks well into old age, because if you don't take care of your skin, melanin-enhanced or not, it will tell on you.

In case you haven't noticed, the emphasis today is on skin care, not exceptional makeup techniques. Those of you who think the depletion of the ozone layer and the increase in incidents of skin cancers worldwide are subjects of interest only to Caucasians should think again. Melanin will protect you longer, but it won't hold up indefinitely, and if you expose your skin long enough, you will eventually damage it. Melanin means you have an *edge,* an *advantage,* but it doesn't mean you have immunity.

Your Skin Anatomy Lesson

Skin is made up of two major sections, the *epidermis* and *dermis.* First things first, starting from the bottom:

THE BOTTOM OF THE BARREL

Underneath everything is a layer of subcutaneous fat, which insulates your body against heat loss and acts as an energy reserve. Heredity and the amount of fat you eat determine how thick this layer is going to be.

SAGGING AND BAGGING SKIN

The next layer—the thickest part of your skin—is called the dermis. The dermis's primary component is collagen, which is the connective protein that gives your skin its support and tautness. Elastin, another fibrous connective found in the dermis, provides elasticity. Elastin allows your skin to stretch without causing immediate and irreversible wrinkles. Both collagen and elastin diminish with age, but genetics and sun damage have a lot to do with how well the skin maintains these two ingredients.

SWEAT, HAIR, AND FUNK

The dermis also contains hair follicles and the sebaceous glands that produce sebum. Sebum is the oily substance that determines whether your skin is dry, oily, or normal. Apocrine glands, located around the genital, anus, and armpits, produce a musky, "funky" sweat. Eccrine glands, located over the entire body, produce the watery, "healthy" sweat. When either of these waste products mix with bacteria on the skin's surface, the result is funk. You now understand why your mother taught you to wash as far as possible and then wash "possible."

THE ICING ON THE CAKE

The epidermis is the topmost layer of skin. It's composed of many layers of cells that are created at the bottom and work their way up to the top layer. Thick skin has many epidermal layers, and thin skin has fewer, but the average skin is only as thick as a sheet of sturdy paper. By the time the cells work their way up to the top layer, they are dead and will slough off naturally (a good part of household dust is, in fact, dead skin cells) or be washed away. Dead cells on top of dark skin tend to have a lighter or ashy cast. Last, but not least, the melanocytes, located in the dermis, produce skin pigment, also known as melanin.

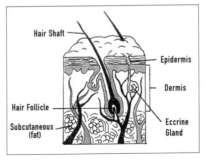

Skin diagram

Black Like Me

Tanning is a Western fashion phenomenon that historically embraced three sentiments: Having a tan meant you could afford to go somewhere warm to get one; tans looked healthy because it meant you were getting your vitamin D from the sun exposure; and (then it got down to vanity) paler skin simply looked more appealing with a bit of color. Before tanning came into vogue, paleness equaled success. In the antebellum South, a magnolia-white complexion was proof positive that you had ladylike breeding and the means—also known as the slaves—to avoid outdoor labor.

Today, many people still like to flaunt a tan, even though it's been revealed to be unhealthy. I know plenty of black people who brag about the tan they got while vacationing in Jamaica. It wasn't that long ago that the idea of a black person pursuing a tan was likened to, say, making your nose wider or your hair nappier, putting a hole in your head, lying down in the middle of the street . . . I think you get the picture.

"Got a min-ute, get a tay-an-n . . . with Coppertone." "Uh, uh, uh," we'd cluck. "Just look at those crazy white folks. Tryin' to get just like us. They wanna be black, but they don't want to *be* black." Yadda, yadda, yadda.

"You don't need to lie out in the sun like that," my mother would say while wondering why my "hardheaded" brother spent so much time in the blazing sun. "Why do you want a tan? You're already a Negro." During the "Black and Proud" era of the seventies, some of our lighter-complexioned black friends would proudly tell us that they had been out in the backyard, roasting in the sun so they could "get black." What they were really getting was sun-damaged skin. Seems like you didn't want to get darker if you were already dark, and getting darker was bad if you weren't that way to begin with.

This is the story on black people and the sun. Sun exposure stimulates the melanocytes, epidermal cells that produce melanin. Racial and genetic makeup determine how much melanin one is born with and how much additional melanin will be produced by sun exposure. People of African descent have the ability to produce more melanin than those of Caucasian descent. Ultraviolet light from sun exposure destroys the elastin and collagen in the skin's dermis layer. In very dark-skinned people the melanin acts as an ultraviolet light filter and protects the elastin and collagen in the dermis from damage. So, even though our melanin filters the UV exposure, the skin has to be exposed to some sun in order to stimulate the melanin. Think of it as damage control. Tanning means that your skin has already had a touch of damage and is tanning in order to prevent more. Many black people

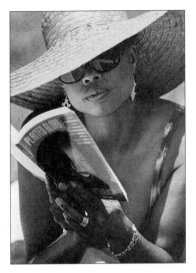

You can be cute and still enjoy the sun. Don't forget to wear sunglasses and sunblock, and to bring along a big shady hat and a good book.

do not equate a tan with sun damage but rather with darkening, which is considered a cosmetic or protective response.

That's where our natural advantage comes in. We already have our melanin UV filter from birth, and because of this, we can be exposed to the sun longer with less damage. Dark-skinned people won't become a mass of wrinkles and sunspots due to one tanning session, but repeated unprotected exposure *will* do you in.

FRECKLES

Skin that freckles is skin that has attempted to produce a brown sheet of melanin but has instead produced isolated spots. This can be caused by genetics and is not uncommon in lighter-complexioned black skin. Melanin production also lessens as you age, so a light-skinned black who didn't freckle in her youth may do so as she gets older.

BLACKBERRIES

The blacker the berry, the sweeter the juice (and if I may add, the prettier the skin). I have seen enough extremely dark-skinned women of a certain age and older with virtually no wrinkling or sagging to conclude that:

A. They had sense enough to stay out of the sun, probably because they already had enough of a good thing.

B. The casual sun exposure that they got was filtered to a fare-thee-well by their naturally dark skin.

You don't have to be a sweet blackberry to remain fine into your old age. If someone were to ask Lena Horne what her beauty secrets are—she reportedly says a face-lift is not one of them—I'm willing to bet that she'd say she avoids the sun.

WILL A TAN LAST FOREVER?

Well, no and yes. The initial tan or extra production of melanin is at the skin's surface until the cells are sloughed away by normal washing. Your tan will also eventually peel away, because the moisture level in the topmost cells is basically nil and your skin is reproducing cells to replace the fried ones. That's the "no" part.

The "yes" part is that tanning equals damage, so at some point you'll see some darkening and/or spotting that doesn't go away. Genetics and the extent of sun damage determine how noticeable this is going to be, which leads to the next question.

GOING DARK IN YOUR OLD AGE

There's nothing sadder than to hear an old person whose complexion is a rich deep chocolate claim that back in the day, they were the color of a young Lena Horne. Who is zooming who? To borrow another lyric from the Queen of Soul, here's the 411: If you are a light-complexioned black person who has worshiped the sun for most of your life, the—yes—accumulated sun damage will cause your skin to darken noticeably as you get older. You don't even have to be a worshiper—just living life without sun protection will be enough to cause some permanent browning and splotchiness. Most accumulated sun damage starts showing up in the late thirties and forties, but it can show up even sooner if your skin is especially sensitive to sunburn. We're not talking about that toasty brown that you got on those vacations to Aruba, either. We're talking about uneven, Leatherette brown with wrinkles and spots. But also understand that we're talking about one or two shades darker than your natural skin color, not a total transformation.

Skin Care and Your Face

Everyone's skin has its own idiosyncrasies, but the general agreement about what makes melanin-enriched skin look its best is pretty basic. The goal is to have an evenly pigmented, or "clear," complexion, fairly small pores, and an absence of zits. If your skin were evenly pigmented with a minimum or absence of blemishes, you'd have a natural foundation, requiring just a dab or so of concealer. Then you could wear foundation only when you really wanted to, not because you can't be seen without it. Sounds simple, but it takes regular maintenance to achieve it. And guess what? Skin care doesn't have to be expensive unless you want it to be.

CLEANSERS

This is the truth about cleansers. Ladies will swear by a certain skin-care line or method, but it's all about your personal preference and skin-care needs. The only people who require certain products are those with serious acne problems. Acne is a condition that requires the expertise of a dermatologist, so before you spend money on over-the-counter remedies, I suggest you see a dermatologist.

Should you use soap and water or a certain cleanser? It really

Tip: You should be more selective about the product that will spend the most time on your skin. This means that cleansers and toners should be the least expensive part of your skin-care regimen. "Least expensive" doesn't mean cheap, it means asking yourself what a $35 cleanser that you rinse or tissue off is going to do for you that a $2.99 cleanser can't. I'm not going to lie here, I like luxury as well as the next woman, but it's good to know about practicalities when the money is tight.

doesn't matter. I've asked women with good skin what they use and some have told me "Ivory and water," while others have said they never use it. Everyone has a different answer. Here's mine. If your skin is oily, it tends to feel cleaner if you use a product that can be rinsed away. Drier skin will usually prefer cleansers that are more emollient, so the skin doesn't feel stripped.

Practicalities

Oatmeal. If you're looking for an extremely affordable cleanser, and one that's widely available, there's no better deal than oatmeal—the same oatmeal you buy at the grocery store. It's tried, it's true, and it works. It is a natural, irritation-free skin cleanser, and is very good for oily skin.

Use regular, old-fashioned oatmeal, not the instant kind.

For a "scrub," use oatmeal straight from the box. Dampen your face and take about a tablespoon of dry oatmeal in your damp hands. Gently work it on your skin in a circular motion. Rinse.

As a cleanser, use it straight from the box or use a blender or mortar and pestle to grind up a half cup of oatmeal into a fine powder. Store the oatmeal in a covered, airtight container—you can recycle sweet-smelling spice jars with screw tops and lids—and keep it in your bathroom. It should last for two months. You'll figure out how much you use each day and can blend up new batches according to your needs.

For a soothing mask, mix oatmeal and plain yogurt into a paste and apply to clean skin. Let it sit for fifteen minutes before rinsing. The oatmeal cleans and soothes and the yogurt tones and lightly exfoliates.

If you like convenience, buy colloidal oatmeal at a drugstore. Colloidal oatmeal is oatmeal that is ground into a fine powder and sold as a bath additive to soothe itchy, irritated skin. The best-known brand name is Aveeno, and their product comes prepackaged; use the "plain" formula, not the moisturizing one. Pour the powder into a plastic shaker-top container and you can shake a little bit into your hands and add water to make a thin paste. Wash your face with it and rinse off. You may find that making masks is easier using colloidal oatmeal.

St. Ives. Let me re-
peat this. St. Ives. This
company makes clean-
sers, moisturizers, and
masks that are very
affordable and avail-
able at drugstores and
supermarkets in most
parts of the country.
They don't skimp on
the amount of product,
and many items come
in tubes handy for
traveling. The jars of
moisturizer and cream

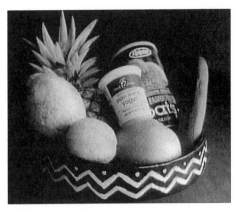

*Affordable, natural skin care. Clockwise from top:
oatmeal, cucumber, grapefruit, lemon, papaya, and
pineapple. Center: yogurt.*

cleanser are so generous that I recommend you don't use your bacte-
ria-laden fingers to scoop out the contents—use a plastic cosmetic
scoop or even a small plastic spoon (that you'll keep clean) and your
product will have a longer shelf life. The cleansers also come in
handy pump dispensers, so you can choose what you like. St. Ives
does try to keep up with the latest trends in skin care, but they seem
to retain the basics, so folks, stay loyal. If you like simple but you
want more than oatmeal, try this line.

Soap. Soap and water have gotten a bad rap because the hype says
soap leaves a film that dries on the skin and causes more problems.
I think part of the hype has a lot to do with the fact that soap
is cheaper than other skin-care products. If you rinse thoroughly and
use a toner, you shouldn't have problems with a soapy film.

Camay and Ivory are established brands. Drier skin may prefer
Tone or Dove.

Clear soaps are good for those concerned about potential irri-
tants—Neutrogena or Pears are two examples.

Oatmeal-based soaps are good for sensitive or irritated skin.

Clinique, a well-established department-store skin-care line, has
an affordable program that consists of a bar of soap, toner, and moisturizer that are keyed to skin type.

Soap-Free Cleansers. A very popular recommendation by doctors for those with sensitive skin. Two examples are Cetaphil and pHisoderm. St. Ives also sells a soap-free cleanser.

Cleansing Creams. Emollient cleansers that are creamed on and tissued/rinsed away, depending upon the formula. Cold creams also fall into this category. The better-known brands are Noxema and Ponds Cold Cream. Albolene cleansing cream is another well-established name.

Oils. You can use oils to break down sebum, dirt, or makeup. Those with acne shouldn't use cleansing oils, but in the case of oily skin, cleansing oil *will* break down skin oils. Sweet Almond Oil is widely available and affordable. If you like luxury, you may want to check out the Clarins skin-care line (available in upscale department stores), which includes wonderfully fragranced botanical oils for cleansing. Smooth a small amount of oil onto dry skin and gently massage it into the skin. Wet a washcloth in *cold* water—this helps lift away the oil more efficiently—and gently wipe away the grime. I didn't think I'd ever use an oil, but now that I live in the land of snow and furnaces, I find that it's one cleanser that won't dry out my skin.

Cleansing Tools

When you wash your face, ideally you remove all traces of cleanser and get a mild exfoliation in the bargain. I find using fingers to be a good idea only if you're cleaning the skin with oatmeal, or applying cleansing grains or scrubs, because your fingers apply them more efficiently than a facial brush or sponge. Try using one of these cleansing aids plus some cotton pads to apply toner.

Gentle Facial Brush. Gentle is the key here. You can find complexion brushes at most beauty supply stores or drugstores. Get the softest natural bristle you can find.

Washcloths. Washcloths develop a layer of dirty makeup mixed with oils or creams. Nothing is less appealing than reaching for a washcloth that is stiff with three days' (and nights') worth of residue. It's better to use a fresh cloth for your face each day. You can use one cloth twice a day, in the morning and at night. Buy packs of cheap white washcloths at your local drug or discount store. Get at least ten, though twice as many is better because then you'll have about a week's worth of extras if you fall behind on the laundry detail. I recommend white because you can throw them in with the rest of your laundry whites and bleach them if you like, plus they make it easier to see how clean you're getting your skin.

Sponges. Organic or synthetic? I prefer organic, and to prevent bacteria and mildew, be sure to rinse them well and dry in a well-ventilated place. To keep organic sponges smelling even sweeter, some users recommend cleaning them in a basin of warm water with a tablespoon of baking soda added to it.

Exfoliating Sponges. The best-known brand is Buf-Puf. I prefer to restrict the use of this to my body, but if you want to use it on your face, I'd recommend using the gentle Buf-Puf with a minimum amount of pressure.

Cotton Pads. I prefer the 100 percent cotton pads that are pressed into round or square pads. Leave the cotton/rayon combos for someone else. Pads are more efficient than cotton balls for applying toner, and one pad will do your whole face and neck (cotton balls are cheaper, but you have to use three or four to do the job of one pad, so where's the savings?). Some people use cotton pads to remove cream cleansers from the face, which doesn't work for me because you have to use several pads to get the job done.

TONERS/ASTRINGENTS

Toners help clear off the remnants of cleanser residue and dirt. They also help refresh and tone the pores. Some dermatologists believe that toners with a high alcohol content strip the skin of its natural sebum coating and the sebaceous glands increase production to compensate for the loss. Toners are not designed to clean your skin, and if you find you're getting a lot of dirt on your cotton pad, your cleansing isn't as thorough as it should be. Remember, you don't want a strong toner because too much alcohol will strip your skin.

Witch hazel is the best product for the best price. You can go with either a brand name or a generic because it's the same thing, but you can usually get the best deal with the large-sized generic bottles. Cooled witch hazel on a cotton pad also soothes tired eyes.

If you prefer a commercial toner, use a mild formula or one for normal skin. Sea Breeze has a toner that's popular, but it contains a high concentration of alcohol. I'd dilute it with water before using it on my face.

If your skin is extremely oily, try an oil-blotting or matte lotion instead of a strong toner. Zero Oil by Origins is a good choice and is available at most department stores. You can use it with or without makeup. Investigate other skin-care/cosmetic lines for similar products.

Note: See the section on skin recipes for toners that you can make yourself for pennies. Always use fresh ingredients because they are the most effective.

Tip: St. Ives makes a good, affordable all-purpose moisturizer.

Tip: If you're inclined to spend a lot on your skin-care regimen, put your money into a moisturizer you like because this is the product that will spend the most time on your skin.

Tip: Eye and neck creams. The skin under your eyes and on your neck is delicate and prone to wrinkling and premature sun damage. You can buy eye and neck creams, but the smarter way to protect these areas is to wear UV-protected sunglasses and use a sunscreen on the neck. At night, gently pat moisturizer around your eye area and massage into your neck.

MOISTURIZERS

Moisturizers are the one item that consistently manage to dumb-found many of us. There are a lot of products on the market and all of them claim to turn back the clock. The truth is that none of them will. The purpose of moisturizer is to create a film or barrier that helps your skin retain whatever natural lipids and moisture it produces on its own. It's a conditioner for the skin; the water-based ingredients hydrate your skin and the emollients help keep the moisture in. That's about it. There are formulas that claim to do more of one than the other, and if you like the way one product feels, then use it.

EXFOLIATORS

Exfoliators have several benefits.

First and foremost, they help the cell-renewal cycle by removing dead skin cells more efficiently, which in turn allows moisturizer to work more efficiently since it is then sealing moisture into living tissue instead of dead skin cells.

Your skin looks better because the "newest" skin is exposed to the surface, and since it is free of ashy patches of dead skin, it looks more evenly toned.

The pore-clogging debris is sloughed away, so you have fewer pimples.

You must exfoliate regularly to enjoy the benefits. When you stop doing it, your skin returns to its previous sluggish, blotchy state. Dermatologists tell me that exfoliating isn't a necessity, but it does work and your skin looks better.

Note: If you're interested in making exfoliators of your own for pennies, see my section on exfoliating mask recipes.

Methods

Manual Exfoliators. A washcloth, Buf-Puf, a complexion brush.

Scrubs or Cleansing Grains. Commercial almond scrubs are the most popular. It's best to use the finest-grained scrub you can because large particles will tear and abrade the skin.

Skin Masks. The tightening effect stimulates the skin, and ingredients like clay help to draw out impurities. The mask tightens and dries, and when you remove it with a wet washcloth, it removes a layer of dead skin cells along with it.

Alpha Hydroxy Acids (AHAs). Sugar, milk, or fruit acids that slough off layers of dead skin cells. Salicylic acid and benzoyl peroxide, which are common ingredients in acne preparations, are also skin sloughers, but they tend to make the skin drier. Enzymes like papain and bromelain (papain is found in papayas, bromelain in pineapples) also slough cells and are a bit gentler than AHAs.

Over-the-counter AHA facial moisturizers, treatments, and cleansers are very efficient exfoliators, but their percentage of acid content is fairly low (generally under 8 percent, or up to 10 percent for "enhanced," over-the-counter preparations), so they must be used almost every day to be effective. AHA products with more than 10 percent acid are usually available directly from an M.D.'s office or licensed skin-care salon. Some AHA facial preparations are AHA/moisturizer combinations. Others are meant to be used with a separate moisturizer.

AHA products for body exfoliation have a slightly higher concentration of acids, so are not recommended for use on the face. But they encourage cell turnover on body sites like the chest and back that are prone to breakouts, and help keep breakouts to a minimum.

Warning: It is not unusual to experience stinging after applying an AHA product, but intense stinging, irritation, or rash are signs that the product is not right for your skin type. You should look for weaker formulations or consult a dermatologist. Before using any AHA product, it isn't a bad idea to patch-test your skin first.

You can overuse AHA products. Dermatologists agree that it is not necessary to use a range of AHA cleanser, toner, moisturizer, foundations, lip creams, and bath gels every day. It isn't necessary to use an AHA cream more than once a day, preferably at night. Use it *after* cleansing and toning the skin but *before* applying moisturizer (unless you use a moisturizer with AHA in it, in which case skip the additional AHA cream). If you do use AHA creams, it is mandatory that you use a sunscreen (most dermatologists recommend at least SPF 15) to prevent hyperpigmentation or photosensitivity.

There are many commercial AHA products available, or you can make a treatment of your own (see the skin recipe section in this book).

How Deep Should You Go?

Dermatologists and many skin-care salons perform AHA and glycolic acid skin peels using products that are not available over the counter. The acid concentration in these products is higher—about 35 to 70 percent—and more effective than what's available in over-the-counter products, but the effects are temporary and the treatments must be repeated regularly in order to maintain the results. Glycolic peels are effective in eliminating sun damage like brown spots, coarsened skin, and superficial wrinkling. A glycolic acid peel removes *surface* skin cells and doesn't result in scarring. Enzyme peels, which use fruit enzymes to remove *dead* skin cells on the skin's surface, are usually safer and not as invasive as the glycolic acid peels, which penetrate the epidermis and remove an epidermal layer. Deep skin peels use trichloroacetic acid, which actually burns off a layer of skin. Deep skin peels and dermabrasion, which physically abrades the skin with fine-grained buffers, are not recommended for dark skin because they could cause blotching and hyperpigmentation. It's best to consult dermatologists and skin salons that are experienced in treating black skin before having a professional glycolic peel.

How to Clean Your Face

1. Remove makeup first. Many commercial skin cleansers will remove makeup, but some of them don't, so read labels carefully before you buy if you want them to do double duty. St. Ives sells a cream cleanser that removes makeup and it's available at most drugstores. Albolene cream will also dissolve makeup—then you can use a damp washcloth to wipe it away. Clinique (available at department stores) sells a makeup solvent in a convenient pump dispenser. If you use the creams or solvents, *always* use a wet washcloth or facial sponge to remove makeup; never use paper tissues on your face, because they are made of wood pulp, which is too rough for your skin.

2. *Apply cleanser.* Use the tool of your choice to apply, and work out the dirt with gentle circular motions, taking care not to stretch the delicate skin around the eyes.

3. *Rinse.* A thorough rinse is the secret to good cleansing.

4. *Dry.* Pat—don't rub—your face dry with a towel. Apply toner with a cotton pad. While face is damp but not dripping, apply moisturizer. If you're applying an alpha hydroxy acid preparation, you should blot your face a bit more before applying because excess water on the skin will dilute the strength of the acid.

5. *Sleep.* Nighttime is rebuild time. In the wee hours of the morning, when traffic is almost nonexistent, it's not uncommon to have transportation workers out on the roads, taking care of business. Your body rebuilds while you are asleep during those same hours, not unlike the road crews. One example of your body's attempt to restore itself can be observed when you go to sleep without cleaning your face and are greeted by a new zit or two the next morning, even if your skin is relatively trouble free. This happens because of cell turnover when the pores and follicles attempt to flush themselves out. They can't do that if the surface of the skin is covered by a sheet of old dead cells, accumulated sebum, and dirt that has settled there from everyday living. Add a layer of stale makeup to this mix and you can also expect to see a little whitehead or blackhead production. After cleansing and toning, all you need to give your skin a good night's rest is a light application of a moisture cream. Coating your face in a mask of cream and sleeping in it is a waste of time and good linens. Take a cue from the road crews: Keep your skin clear while you sleep so your body can get some work done.

Skin-Care Specialists

Some of you may want something a bit more indulgent than a home-made papaya mask, and so you may want to check out an esthetician, also known as a skin-care specialist. It's worth the bucks to go to salons that have first-class reputations for pampering. I am referring to salons or people who perform skin-care services, not people who use "home facial parties" to sell cosmetic products. The people wearing the white coats at the cosmetic counters offering facials are not estheticians, they are salespeople.

Many skin-care salons offer facials, superficial acid and enzyme peels, massage, skin extractions, manicures and pedicures, body wraps, and salt scrubs. Some offer hairdressing services as well, but I've found that the skin-care salons that concentrate on skin care are usually your best bet.

First, the facialist will ask about your skin-care regimen, examine your skin, and ask what services you want if you haven't already specified them. Then your skin is steamed (the steaming continues throughout the facial), makeup is removed, and the skin is cleansed and lightly massaged. At some point the facialist will per-form a skin extraction—that is, squeezing and removing blackheads or pimples that have come to a head. You are usually asked if you have a strenuous objection to this, because it's slightly uncomfort-able, but it is worth the trouble. Then a soothing mask is applied. When the facial is over, some salons let you know what products they use in case you want to purchase any of them. Others leave it up to you to ask. It's customary to tip the facialist 10 to 15 percent of the price of the facial. Usually, your skin feels so clean and smooth that you hate to put makeup on afterward, and it's actually better if you let it breathe at least until the next day.

I've sampled several skin-care salons, including one that caters to a black clientele, one that specializes in botanical products, one that caters to the well-heeled and the well-known, and one that has branches in major cities. If you've never had a professional facial and you want to start, try the Elizabeth Arden Salon, which has locations in most major cities. Here are some things you should be aware of:

THE QUALIFICATIONS

Miss Edith or Mr. Paul should be a state-licensed esthetician/skin-care professional at the bare minimum. A professional trained in skin care is not equal to a dermatologist, who is a medical doctor, though there are many estheticians, such as clinical estheticians with advanced training, who work with dermatologists. The basic training for a skin-care professional can be obtained at most cosmetology schools. Any procedure that involves an injection should be administered by a physician.

THE AMBIANCE

My feeling is this: I want a high quotient of luxury and pampering.

I don't want to wait more than fifteen minutes in the waiting area. At the better salons, I barely had time to thumb through a magazine before someone whisked me off to have my facial.

I want soothing music played low, and other than telling me what she is putting on my skin, I want the esthetician to keep the talking to a minimum. Her job is to put me at ease, not necessarily to relate what's going on in her life in great detail. Of course, if you prefer small talk, ask a few questions, but the esthetician should leave that option up to you.

The salon should be clean and a smock should be supplied to protect your clothing.

Know the difference between a skin-care salon and a skin clinic that emphasizes corrective services. Corrective clinics may not offer the luxurious ambiance that you associate with a facial salon, but the fee may be lower. You may not get the soothing face and neck massage, the calming music, or even a gown to change into. The esthetician may interrupt your appointment to tend to some other business. And don't count on leaving a skin clinic feeling relaxed and pampered. At one of these clinics that I visited, the little cubicles had curtains that were a perfect conduit for hearing more than I ever wanted to know about someone else's business. During my facial, I overheard the woman in the next cubicle telling the heartbreaking and grisly story of how her son was hit by a train. If you are paying $45 to $70 for a facial, you may prefer to be in your own little room with your very own facialist giving you 100 percent of her attention.

THE SALES PITCH

There is nothing wrong with a facialist telling you what she is applying during the course of the facial, but the better salons won't take it any further than that, because if you're crazy about a certain product, you're going to ask for it on your own. Some facialists prefer not to divulge any of their secrets and I can understand why. I tried asking what one facialist was using on me and she told me that all the products she used were only available to professional estheticians. I think you have to decide why you're going for a professional facial in the first place: You want the pampering done by someone else (otherwise, you'd go to a beauty supply store and buy your own mud mask). Some skin-care salons offer their own product line to customers, but this is not unlike hairdressers who sell shampoo and conditioners. Their primary income should be derived from performing services, not selling products.

Beware: If you have a real problem with your skin and substitute a skin-care salon for a medical professional, then you're going in for an expensive and probably ineffective solution. My personal experience has been that if you hear the word *acne* being used to describe your skin condition, then the word *dermatologist* should follow somewhere in the conversation. If the dermatologist recommends that you get serviced by a clinical esthetician, that's fine and perhaps your medical insurance can pick up some of the cost. One salon recommended I buy their $250 to $300 skin-maintenance program to help clear up my "acne" skin condition. I didn't want to spend that kind of money, so I purchased the benzoyl peroxide and sulfur soap they recommended, which cost $70. That ain't cheap, the products weren't effective on my skin condition, and I still didn't know what the problem was. For the $70 I could have seen a dermatologist and nailed down the problem.

Dermatologists

So you hear the word *acne* and you need a dermatologist—where should you find one? First look for a dermatologist who is highly experienced in dealing with black skin. Ask around and do your homework. Cities with large black populations as well as large university centers, teaching hospitals, and medical schools are good places to seek dermatologists with the expertise you need or to find leads to ones who are qualified.

MOLE REMOVAL

Nigra papulosa, the flat brown or little moles that stick up on the face, are common in people of African descent. They usually crop up around the eyes and on the cheeks (as well as on the chest). They're harmless but sometimes cosmetically undesirable. They run in my family, and a friend once told me to tie a thread around the stem of the mole and it would drop off. It worked, but the mole soon began to come back. Dermatologists advise against this because of the possibility of infection. A doctor can remove them easily using a mild acid, or by freezing or burning them off.

SKIN TAGS

These are flesh-colored growths that stick out from the skin like little tags. They are commonly found around the neck, waist, or underarms, areas usually subject to friction from clothing. One home cure for these is to tie a horse hair around the base. Interesting, but the dermatologist can take care of these as well. Skin tags are harmless, but if they occur in an area of the body that is subject to constant rubbing, they can become irritated and bleed.

KELOID REMOVAL

Keloids, or raised scars, are common in people of African descent. Keloids can develop wherever the skin has been cut or on sites where the skin has been pierced. A dermatologist can minimize or remove excess scar tissue. The tendency to develop keloids is inherited, so if you are prone to them, think twice before going in for cosmetic surgery or body piercing.

ACNE TREATMENT

Severe acne eruptions are commonly treated by dermatologists. Over-the-counter remedies may help for minor outbreaks, but black skin has a tendency toward hyperpigmentation, so it is probably better to seek professional help.

RASH TREATMENT

Reddened, weeping, or encrusted rashes, such as psoriasis or impetigo, should be examined by a dermatologist.

VITILIGO TREATMENT

Vitiligo is the condition that entertainer Michael Jackson made famous. It affects the melanocytes, which in this case stop producing pigment. This is not limited to people of African descent, it is simply more noticeable in them because of the obvious pigment contrast. The spots commonly begin occurring around body orifices. Medical experts aren't sure why this occurs, though one recent theory is that it's the result of a virus. Dermatologists are currently treating vitiligo with the drugs Psoralin and Benoquin, and using ultraviolet light to restore melanin production. This is not a condition to play around with. If you see unusual-looking pale spots that have gradually enlarged, see a dermatologist.

RETIN-A

Retin-A received a whole lot of press as the "youth" cream of the eighties. It is a derivative of vitamin A and was originally used to treat acne, but in the late eighties a doctor noted that it also reversed the effects of sun-damaged skin and people went wild. The word is that it is supposed to boost production of elastin and collagen as well as accelerate cell turnover, which lightens and "repairs" sun-damaged skin. It all sounds good, but there's always a downside.

Many women who take Retin-A experience considerable burning, itching, and peeling and generally have to go through a period of adjustment before their dermatologist figures out the concentration with the least irritation factor. A low concentration isn't always effective.

Because of the increased skin sensitivity, Retin-A users are advised to use specific cleansers and moisturizers, and you can be sure that these are not dollar-days bargains.

Once you start a Retin-A regimen, it thins and photosensitizes the skin, so you must *always* use a sunblock of at least SPF 15 for-ever after or your skin will darken and spot. Retin-A is currently available by prescription only, which means it isn't cheap, and once you stop using it, all the same old problems will return. But caveats aside, if you have severe acne or sun-damaged skin, Retin-A may be a good bet.

RENOVA

Renova is a wrinkle cream containing tretinoin, a vitamin A deriva-tive. Tretinoin penetrates the epidermal layer to remove skin cells, which irritates the dermis. Irritation means burning, stinging, or peeling. According to the product description, the cell turnover stimulates collagen production and decreases wrinkles and brown spots. Because the cream penetrates the dermal layer, there is a warning about its safety and effectiveness for people with moderately or heavily pigmented skin. It doesn't repair sun damage; in fact, it heightens sun sensitivity, and sunblock must be worn while using it. A prescriptive treatment, Renova has to be used for a minimum of six months in order to achieve results.

How to Allow Yourself to Be Seen Without Makeup

Clear skin means, ideally, your shade of brown with no dark spots or blotches. There are several ways to help this along.

DRINK PLENTY OF WATER

Yes, the eight-glasses-a-day rule is true. I used to ignore it and then I noticed that my skin looked a lot better after a short vacation in an extremely hot climate. Why? Because I was consuming a minimum of eight glasses a day and my body was able to flush itself of impuri-ties. Ever notice how your breath smells when you haven't been drinking enough water? How your perspiration goes from a healthy sweat to a malodorous one? Or how skin eruptions seem to prolifer-ate? Water plays a major part in your skin's ability to eliminate wastes. Try drinking a *minimum* of eight glasses a day for four days and notice the difference in your skin.

EXFOLIATE REGULARLY

As you age, your cell turnover slows down. The dead skin cells accumulate in uneven spots and that causes some areas of your skin to appear darker or blotchier than others. You must help the cycle along by sloughing away dead skin cells. Use a complexion brush, skin scrubs, or fruit acid exfoliants like a papaya enzyme mask.

AVOID PICKING YOUR FACE

Picking pimples before they're ready to erupt on their own breaks the skin, and the trauma causes skin to darken around the spot. Use commercial preparations containing salicylic acid or benzoyl peroxide to encourage the skin on the pimple to slough off, which then exposes the pus or sebum and helps you to remove it by *gently* pressing, then washing with a washcloth. Check out the acne preparations on the market. Many formulations come in stick form so you can dab it on isolated pimples. This is recommended if you have occasional flare-ups or pimples, but if you have severe acne, you should see a dermatologist.

REMOVE BLACKHEADS GENTLY

Blackheads are pores that are clogged with a plug of darkened sebum. If the plug is not dislodged during normal cleansing, you should remove it. Steaming the skin, which opens the pores, makes removal easier. Use a blackhead extractor, which is a small metal tool with holes on either end that allows you to press the area around the blackhead without damaging the skin and causing a dark spot. Blackhead extractors are available at drugstores and beauty supply stores (this is what estheticians use during the "extraction" portion of your facial).

If you can't resist picking your face and you get dark spots, use fade cream to fade the dark spot *only*. Remember, you want the dark spot to fade back to your natural color.

USE SUNSCREEN

If you use fade creams or lotions, also be sure to use sunscreen because the newly lightened skin will be sensitive to the sun and exposure will cause a reactive development of melanin, which will darken the same spot.

Wantu Wazuri Use Bleaching Cream

Artra, Nadinola, Black and White Cream. I remember my grandmother Phronie's beauty basics were her Watermelon lipstick, her black hair dye, Mum deodorant, and Nadinola, "to keep her complexion clear." I wasn't about to argue with that. When my zits came in, along with the dark spots from picking them, my mom gave me some Noxzema to wash with and Artra to bring my skin back. I must have been the last person alive who actually believed that stuff about fading spots caused by pimples and blackheads. Apparently, there were a lot of people who were using fade creams to get a "clear" complexion. My aunt told me that she went to high school with several girls whose faces were clearly three shades lighter than their necks, hands, and the rest of their bodies, the results of fade cream abuse. When dermatologist Paul Kelley told me that folks have been known to bathe in a bathtub of Clorox bleach, in the belief that they would become lighter, I almost fell out of my chair. It makes my skin feel raw and blistered just thinking about that one.

THE SMART WAY TO FADE

Hyperpigmentation or overproduction of melanin due to trauma is a common problem with dark skin. The smart way to use fade creams is to use them to fade *dark spots only*. The idea is to maintain evenly pigmented skin by helping the overpigmented areas fade back to their normal pigment, not to change the color you were born with.

Fade creams or lotions contain about 2 percent hydroquinone, which removes melanin. Because of this, you should always use a sunblock to prevent the same area from darkening again. If you apply fade creams at night, you won't have to worry about immediate sun exposure, but you should continue to wear sunscreen during the day. Those on the go may want to consider Fashion Fair Cosmetics' fade cream, which is combined with sunscreen. I use Black Opal Dual Action Fade Gel on my spots if I can't wait for them to fade naturally. This brand combines hydroquinone with an alpha hydroxy acid to slough away old skin cells so that the hydroquinone works more effectively.

Fade creams aren't always necessary to banish spots caused by skin eruptions. If you can wait it out without picking the blemish, most dark spots will fade by themselves. Remember that this works only if the blemish hasn't been picked into a major crater.

Shave and a Haircut, Two Bits

We've all seen ladies of a certain age with a mustache and goatee that a thirteen-year-old boy would envy. My reaction has always been "Isn't she going to *do* something about that?" I'm sure I'm not the only one asking, either. I've been told that some men find a mustache (goatee, sideburns) attractive on a woman, which I find hard to believe. I've also been told that it is a generational thing, that some women let things grow wild because they fear shaving will backfire on them—you know, the old chestnut about shaving causing hairs to come back thicker and stronger. If this was the case, I'd just as soon risk the backfire. Still other women have simply thrown in the towel after a certain age and let Nature do whatever she will because they have more pressing things to worry about. Whatever.

There are some legitimate concerns here. People of African descent with tightly coiled hair are more prone to developing ingrown hairs, where the hair curls back on itself and grows into the skin, causing inflamed bumps. We've all seen men struggle with razor bumps and rashes, so the idea of fooling around with the hair on our faces is no small concern. However, because we are female, the heaviness and amount of our facial hair is usually nowhere near what men have. It is common to see a softer, downier variety in our younger years, and as we age and go through hormonal changes, it becomes wirier. That's why the classic bearded lady is the exception rather than the rule.

GETTING RID OF THE BEARD

It's a good idea to get rid of stray hairs when they begin to appear. A general rule to remember is that consistent removal of the hair will weaken the hair follicle so that it will either grow in weaker or die altogether.

Plucking

This is practical if you have a few stray hairs to remove, as in the beginnings of a beard or mustache. Ice the area to soothe it before you pluck. Use tweezers to grab the base of the hair firmly so that you'll remove the entire hair by the root, or you'll end up with hyperpigmented dark spots from ingrown hairs, which will compound your problems. Spend a couple extra dollars for precision tweezers—it's worth it. I recommend using tweezers manufactured by a company called Tweezerman; they're available at your local beauty supply store and most drugstores.

Pumicing

Pumicing the hair or gently abrading it away with a pumice stone or large, flat emery-type board is an old method of removing the hair. It may work for some, but it I find it too easy to miss the hair and abrade the skin. This is also not desirable for dark-skinned women who may have a tendency toward hyperpigmentation.

Shaving

This is a big no-no. A razor on your legs is okay, a razor anywhere on your face is not. This includes eyebrows, sideburns, or anywhere. Leave it for the men. Can you imagine explaining razor burn or shaving nicks?

Depilatories

These are creams, lotions, or foams with a chemical that gently dissolves hair at the base of the root.

Pro: They are pretty effective when used correctly.

Con: Depilatories don't last as long as waxing. They take several minutes to use, and if your application isn't even and the hairs don't disintegrate completely enough, you may have some stray hairs, and to prevent irritation you won't be able to shave for at least twenty-four hours. Depilatories also tend to have a lingering stink, so this is not something to use at the last minute before a date comes to pick you up.

Important: Be sure to patch-test a depilatory before using it, *especially* if it's intended to remove facial hair. This is extremely important; some black men have tried to avoid razor bumps (curly ingrown hairs) by using a well-known shaving depilatory, only to end up with a beard-shaped rash because they were sensitive to the product's ingredients. Don't use facial depilatories intended for male facial hair on your face. And don't substitute products designed to remove leg and underarm hair for facial depilatories, either.

Waxing

Melted wax is applied by a spatula or roller applicator to the hairy area and a strip of cloth or flexible paper is smoothed on top of the site while the wax is still warm. When the wax cools, the paper/cloth is stripped away and the hair, embedded in the cooled wax, comes out by the root.

Pro: This can be very effective for those with sideburns, mustaches, and goatees. Waxing is also effective in removing excess hair from the legs and bikini line, and if you're plagued with ingrown underarm hairs, it can be used there as well. If done professionally, you get a smooth, hairless look that plucking just doesn't beat. The hair takes weeks to grow back, and repeated waxing weakens the roots. In time, the hair will be much lighter and maybe even pluckable.

Con: You'll have to let the hair grow in a little bit so that it will be long enough to catch in the wax strips. You can bleach the stubble if you're light skinned, though I don't know how this goes over with darker skin. And yes, waxing stings, but it's over quickly.

You can have a professional do the job for you, which I recommend if you have a lot of hair to remove, or you can buy a waxing kit at your beauty supply store and do it yourself. If you're a novice do-it-yourselfer, I'd start with the roll-on waxing kits that come with a warming unit and roll-on applicators. The cold waxing kits, which contain strips of paper coated with an extremely sticky wax (sort of like human flypaper), aren't as effective as the hot methods.

Electrolysis

The electrolysist inserts a thin needle into your hair follicles to destroy the roots with small amounts of electric current. This works for some people some of the time. If the hair is zapped enough times, it dies, but the electrolysist has to find the same hair to zap repeatedly, which means it's a hit-or-miss situation. It's also not the cheapest way to go, and if you don't like pain, you won't like electrolysis. The women I know who've had this have quit doing it. I'd consider this as a last resort. If you're thinking of electrolysis, get personal recommendations and find a licensed electrolysist.

Laser Hair Removal

This is a recent development in the follicle war. Be warned that it isn't cheap, but the results sound very promising, especially for the hirsute woman. A laser is used to destroy the hair follicles; like electrolysis, this takes more than one treatment, but the results seem to be more successful. Ideally, laser treatments should catch the hairs in their anagen, or growing phase, when the follicle is at its largest and can be kept from producing more hair. The hairy area is waxed to remove visible hair and rubbed with carbon lotion to soak the hair follicles. A laser is then moved over the lotioned skin, which absorbs the laser light, destroying the hair follicles. Reportedly, it feels like a hot, intense shower. Three treatments are recommended, and the results are said to be much better and longer lasting than waxing or electrolysis.

The War on Ashiness

IDENTIFYING THE ENEMY

Skin sloughs off a layer of dead, dry cells. Since these cells are indeed lifeless and desiccated, their melanin content is basically nil. When you place a thin layer of grayish cells against a light complexion, the skin appears dry or dull with yellowish patches. Take the same layer of dead cells and place them on top of a darker complexion and the contrast is obvious. The skin looks ashy.

It seems that a lot of my formative skin-care days were spent applying lotion in the never-ending War on Ashiness. I never thought the lotion companies were serious about moving product, because if they were, they wouldn't have run those ads about the "soothing properties" of lotion. Black people didn't care about the "moisturizing" qualities in a lotion. We didn't care about the healing properties of aloe. We didn't care that you could pour some lotion on a dried-out leaf and have it spring back green and supple. We bought lotion because it got rid of that *ash*!

One had to be careful with lotions because going cheap was sure to backfire on you at the most inopportune moment. Most people I knew stuck with the tried-and-true standbys, Jergens and Vaseline Intensive Care, which were widely available and affordable. When a company came out with a formula that really held the ash, then you'd see it stocked in folks' bathrooms, and the brand name would spread from household to household. If you saw someone's bathroom shelf stocked with a generic or no-name dollar-days brand, then chances were good that they went cheap and were now walking around ashy. Those weak "moisturizing" lotions worked for about an hour before the ash sprang back up. Doubling up on the amount didn't work, because then you'd spend twenty minutes trying to massage the lotion into your legs—and you'd still be ashy an hour later (except it was worse this time because you'd gone ahead and left the house wearing a sleeveless top and shorts, since you thought you'd lotioned up good that morning).

How to Win the Skirmish

If you want your skin to glow, you've got to get rid of the dead, scaly cells. Greasing and oiling and lotioning them to death doesn't work because then you've got a layer of oil mixed with the dead cells, and when the oils or creams wear away, the ashy cells tend to stick around. The smart way is to exfoliate, or remove as much of the scale as possible, so you won't waste that Vaseline. For more detailed methods, see this chapter's section on bathing.

If you're reading this section with interest, then you probably know that scrubbing and over-the-counter bleaching creams alone are pretty much worthless when it comes to darkened knees and elbows. Here are some other things to try:

Alpha Hydroxy Creams and Lotions

These will do a more efficient job of exfoliating the dead and darkened skin. Two widely available names are Alpha Hydrox, which makes a body cream and a lotion (choose the formula with the higher concentration—10 percent—of acid), and Black Opal, which makes an AHA treatment called Retexturizing Complex. You may want to investigate other lines as well.

Skin-Care Salons

They may offer glycolic acid peels and treatments and creams with a slightly higher concentration of AHAs. The creams are products that you will probably want to purchase for home use.

Dermatologists

They may offer skin-lightening treatments that include a combination of hydroquinone and kojic acid. Kojic acid is derived from mushrooms and is not as invasive as the "deep" peeling acids. It is mostly available through dermatologists, but I've visited at least one skin-care salon that offered treatments using it.

Protect Knees and Elbows

Leaning on the elbows encourages darkening and callusing. If you have to be down on your knees, use knee pads or a soft towel or cushion. (Remember, if your legs are to be exposed to the sun for long periods of time, use a sunblock on the areas you've lightened, because the AHAs and lightening agents will make those areas prone to darkening again.)

The Vaseline Story

People have been bragging about the virtues of Vaseline as a "youth-enhancing moisturizer," but I only knew it as the A-bomb in the War

on Ashiness, the cure for ashy legs across the Diaspora. Lotion was a luxury that was a little too easy to waste. I knew kids who would run from a jar of Vaseline but would try to bathe in a bottle of Jergens. Some even made a game out of putting it on: You could pump out lines of dots along your arms and legs or write your name on your thigh. When you slipped up and ran out of lotion, the most you could do was turn the bottle upside down and catch the last drops. But *nobody* ever ran out of Vaseline. Everyone knew how far you could stretch a jumbo-sized jar of Vaseline. A jar that appeared to be empty could sit in the bathroom for several weeks, and not a soul in the house would go out ashy. That's because folks knew how to get every last bit from every nook and cranny of the jar, including the rim and the screw top. And if the nooks and crannies were cleaned out, you could take a tissue and wipe the entire inside of the jar and be rewarded with enough Vaseline to go outside wearing slingbacks. By that time, somebody would have picked up some Jergens and another jar of Vaseline.

Yes, Vaseline was a guaranteed ash remedy, but some of us were too refined to go public about it. It was more middle class to pour lotion from a bottle of Vaseline Intensive Care than to scoop out a handful of Vaseline. But when the lotion was gone, that "refinement" was thrown out the window, like when it was time to go to church. Legs shining, faces beaming—it went beyond mere cosmetics. Racial pride was at stake here, and there were plenty of mothers who openly declared that they didn't care if "folks have to wear shades when they look at you in church or if your legs are so greasy that you slide off the pew. I'm not having any child of mine walking around looking like somebody's orphan!" In the black community, orphan starts with an *A*, and *A* stands for *ash.*

So now that people have sworn to the virtues of Vaseline as a beauty aid, I had to get the lowdown on it.

When I appeared on *Oprah* to promote my first book, *Good Hair*, the male makeup artist who did me up (and let me tell you, the man is gifted with skills) had gorgeous skin and I asked him what he used.

"Vaseline, honey. I use it every night. Got it from my grandmother."

I have heard variations of the Vaseline story over and over again.

At the African Marketplace Festival in Brooklyn one time, I saw a mature, deep-chocolate-skinned woman who was marketing skin-care products. When I say "mature," I'm saying she was older than me, but I knew she didn't look anywhere near her true age. I asked about her skin. She told me she couldn't lie, it had nothing to do with the skin-care line. It was genetics and Vaseline every night. If I thought my skin would look as good as hers did, I'd *eat* a teaspoon of Vaseline every night.

My friend Dianne swears by a combo of Vaseline and baby oil for smooth, ash-free skin. My aunt Hattie scoped out my rusty heels in a pair of sandals one Sunday morning and advised me that "a little Vaseline would hold them."

I'd always thought that Vaseline or petroleum jelly was far too greasy and thick to be used on the face, that one would end up with a face full of zits. So I asked a few dermatologists who have a predominantly black patient base what they thought about this. They agreed that moisturizing the face with petroleum jelly might not be everyone's cup of tea, but so many people use it to moisturize the body that it is probably a safe bet to use it on your face if you don't mind the texture. At any rate, a little dab will probably do it for you. Get the jumbo-sized jar.

Bathing

In my family, there were two methods of bathing the young ones: a wash-up in the morning ("Wash your face, underarms, and as far as possible, and then wash 'possible'") and a bath at night. I don't believe this was about water conservation as much as it was about keeping the water bill low. A shower was a special treat for us and we wanted it to last until the hot-water tank was empty. This was not such a treat for my mother, who had the task of repairing my frizzed-up press-and-curl after my shower party was over.

Since I was brought up as a tub bather, it naturally followed that as soon as I was permitted, I jumped into the shower and left those time-consuming baths in the dust. It was quite a while before I came back home to the tub, but when I did I rediscovered all sorts of benefits. I hope you will, too.

POLISHING YOUR BODY

The most valuable skin-care lesson my mother taught me about bathing involved scrubbing. She used a surgical scrub brush that she brought home twenty-five years ago. I can still remember the sound of my brother splashing and squalling in the tub as my mother went to work with the scrub brush. One of her pet peeves was seeing a ring of dirt around the back of the neck, and he was usually guilty of this. Well, she still has the brush and she still uses it. It is made of ivory-colored plastic with black nylon bristles and fits into the palm of the hand. I know that natural bristles are the thing now, but I'll tell you that the one my mother has is a great little brush. I've tried to swipe this brush in recent years and have been busted before I could get out of her bathroom. My mother's skin has always been flawless and she has always touted the benefits of a good scrub.

My mother introduced me to the basics of exfoliation, and her sister Martha put the finer points on it. Like my mother, Martha inherited the Blanding skin—chocolate brown, smooth, and pore-less. Woe to those who disparage dark skin, because this is the skin that endures while the rest of us wrinkle and spot our way into old age. Martha worked out with the loofah and pumice long before I knew what the deal was. And unlike some dark-skinned women who are plagued with ash, I can honestly say that I can't ever remember seeing my mother or Martha with ashy skin.

Using a mere washcloth on the body simply doesn't exfoliate as well as a good scrubbing. I like to think of it as polishing the skin, because once the dead cells have been removed and the body is moisturized, dark skin gleams. Ironically, scrubbing is so efficient at lifting the grime and ash that it drove me away from tub bathing when I was young. As a child, seeing the grayish film of dirt floating around the edges of the bathwater and having to clean the ring of scum off the tub pretty much evaporated the allure of tub bathing. What was the point of adding bath salts or bubble bath if it was all going to be grimed away?

Here is a tip that will make bathing more enjoyable: Exfoliate and shower away the grime *before* getting into the tub. Your bath additives will be more effective and you'll have less of a mess to clean up.

Exfoliators

Bath specialty stores and boutiques like The Body Shop have become very popular lately and offer a variety of body-pampering items. Nowadays, you can even find bath accessories in your local supermarket. There are many cultures that use bathing—and have for centuries—as a ritual for socializing, as well as a means of caring for the body. Keep this in mind when you travel, so you can pick up a unique collection of bathing accessories. In the meantime, here are some accessories that you can find in your area.

Loofah. A loofah is a piece of dried gourd that is quite efficient at exfoliating the skin. You can get little loofah mitts and back scrubbers at bath shops and drugstores. You can also grow your own in the backyard (see the skin-care recipes for easy instructions on how to do it). To prolong its use and keep it fresh, be sure to shake out excess water and let it dry after scrubbing.

Scrub Brush. Your best selection will probably be in the bath specialty stores. Natural bristles are best. You may want to get a complexion brush, long-handled back scrubber, and a shorter-handled body brush. These must also be allowed to dry between scrubbings or the bristles will mildew and shed.

Body Buf-Puf. If you're used to a washcloth, then please use this with a gentle hand until your skin has become accustomed to it. Don't confuse the body Buf-Puf with the one for your face. I find that the rougher (blue) side of the body Buf-Puf is very efficient at exfoliating, and once you become accustomed to it, you can use it every day. Your skin will be very smooth and polished and you'll notice a drastic reduction in flaky skin.

Net Scrubber. This nylon net "flower" is very popular now and you can get it just about everywhere. You can also make your own with nylon netting from a fabric store. You will find that a net scrubber is a step above a washcloth, and while it won't do as good a job as other methods, it's good to use between your regular exfoliation sessions.

Scrubbing Glove or Mitt. These nubby-textured items are becoming popular and are a step above net scrubbers in abrasiveness. They are efficient because you can apply even pressure by design, but they won't substitute for a good scrub brush, Buf-Puf, or loofah.

Pumice Stone. Pumice is a porous volcanic stone used to remove calluses from the heels and soles of the feet. It lasts a long time but must be allowed to drain and air frequently or it will become slimy and mildewed.

Rough Grit Foot-Polishing Paddle. I prefer this to the pumice stone. One side has a rough grit to take off the roughened heel skin, while the side with the smoother grit smoothes and polishes. Keep one in the bathroom and make it part of your regimen and you won't be caught with rough, dry calluses.

Nail Brush. These are very cheap and you can get them in all kinds of whimsical shapes. Keep one by the sink and one in your bath and shower. You don't have to stick to natural bristles for this brush.

Sea Salt (or Use Epsom or Kosher Salt). Salt scrubs are great exfoliators. You'll use cups of it at a time, so buy large quantities at the cheapest prices. The best deal on sea salt is usually at your health store or natural food market, where it is often sold by the pound. Kosher salt can be found at your local supermarket in large boxes.

Commercially Prepared Body Scrubs. The most popular of these are the almond or apricot pit scrubs. Get the largest quantity you can because

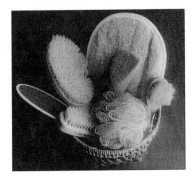

Skin sloughers and smoothers. Clockwise from top: loofah pad, complexion brush, net scrubber, nail brush, callus paddle file, bath brush, and pumice.

you'll use a lot of it. Don't scrimp on the quality; you don't want huge grains because they damage your skin.

Exfoliation Techniques

Dry Scrub. Before you wet your body, loosen the dead skin with the loofah, scrub brush, or Buf-Puf, then scrub your body all over using firm strokes. Wash off the residue in the shower and get into the tub.

Salt Scrub. Mix together baby oil and enough large-grained salt (sea, Epsom, or kosher) to make a paste. Rub the paste all over your body in a circular motion, paying special attention to your elbows, knees, and rough spots. Rinse off in the shower, wash with shower gel, and hop into the tub.

Body Masks. You can use a homemade mask or a commercial preparation. You can adapt the face mask recipes to use as body masks—just double or triple the amount of ingredients.

If your chest (the area above your breasts) and back are prone to breakouts, try the clay mask after exfoliating.

Treat your breasts to a soothing yogurt, honey, or avocado mask. Exfoliate first before applying the mask. Rinse and moisturize your body.

BATH ADDITIVES

Try adding one of these to tepid (body temperature) or very warm bathwater.

Sea Salt

The salt bath is soothing and relaxing and helps condition the skin. Add three cups of salt (sea or kosher) to a tub of warm water.

Seaweed

You can buy powdered seaweed at health stores or allow dried seaweed to soak in a very warm tub for a few minutes to release the benefits. If you use dried seaweed, try tying it in a piece of gauze before soaking or you'll have to take care that it doesn't clog up the drain. After you've soaked in the tub for a while, you can scrub your skin with the gauze-wrapped seaweed, which will serve as a toner. Seaweed helps deep-clean and eliminate toxins, as well as soothes sunburn. You can also mix powdered seaweed with the salt bath.

Baking Soda

Baking soda softens the skin. Mix a quarter cup of baking soda into a warm tub.

Oatmeal

Oatmeal is a natural cleanser that softens and soothes irritated skin. Add a package of colloidal oatmeal (try Aveeno) or a cup of finely ground oatmeal.

Milk

Milk is a good skin softener. Add one or two packets of dried milk to a warm tub.

Cider or Wine Vinegar

Both soften and tone the skin. They also soothe sore muscles. Add two to three cups of vinegar to a warm bath.

Rice Wine

It helps eliminate toxins and tone the skin. Buy a large, cheap bottle of rice wine and pour the whole bottle into the bath.

Oils

Use lavender for relaxation and any of the citrus essences for invigoration. Add anywhere from a few drops to a teaspoon to a warm tub.

Fresh Crushed Mint Leaves

Mint refreshes and invigorates. Add a handful under running water.

Crushed Sprigs of Fresh Rosemary

Rosemary is naturally astringent and good for oily skin. You can also add a teaspoon of rosemary oil to your bath water. The scent is pungent but invigorating.

Fresh Rose Petals

The rose petals are fragrant as well as soothing to dry skin.

BATH TEMPERATURE

It's best to keep the bath comfortably warm because very hot baths can damage your capillaries, which contributes to spider veins. Soaking in very hot baths for too long will dry out your skin and make you dizzy. It's a good idea to have a glass of cool water, herbal tea, or juice nearby before you begin your soak.

NATURAL SKIN-CARE RECIPES

Making your own cosmetic products doesn't have to be a labor-intensive process, and it doesn't mean you have to spend long hours tracking down exotic ingredients. I became interested in skin-care recipes because I noticed organic ingredients and botanical essences had become a big business. Check out the fact that many of the expensive wrinkle creams—Retin-A, Renova, and the alpha hydroxy acids—involve some sort of cell-sloughing accelerator, which can be derived from fruits or vegetables. An enzyme peel at a facial salon may cost you thirty-five dollars, but you can buy a fresh papaya and a pineapple—which contain the same enzymes found in the commercial peels—for five dollars or less if you live where they grow in abundance.

Natural skin-care recipes can be traded with your friends and altered to your liking. You never have to worry about your product going out of fashion or out of production. If you run out of a commercial preparation, you can go to the kitchen or garden and whip something up.

Cleansers

Oatmeal Cleanser or Scrub

½ cup colloidal or finely ground oatmeal

Use a blender or mortar and pestle to grind up a half cup of oatmeal into a fine powder. Store in a covered container—you can recycle sweet-smelling spice jars with screw tops and lids—and keep in your bathroom. Store the oatmeal in an airtight container and it should last for two months. You can blend up new batches according to your needs.

Mix oatmeal with enough water to make a paste and apply to the skin in a circular motion. Rinse off with warm water, then apply toner and moisturizer.

If you want more exfoliation (as a scrub), use oatmeal straight from the box and wet your skin before applying, then rinse off and continue skin regimen.

Yogurt Cleanser

This is good for normal skin.

1 teaspoonful of yogurt
1 teaspoonful of fresh lemon juice (don't use reconstituted lemon juice)

Mix ingredients together and apply to your face. Rinse off with warm water and apply toner and moisturizer. Mix up fresh for each cleansing.

Enzyme Exfoliators

Important: Some skin is more sensitive than others, so if your skin begins stinging unbearably when using the enzyme masks, please rinse it off. You can use plain yogurt to soothe your skin.

Papaya Enzyme Mask

1 ripe papaya
1/4 cup of plain yogurt

Peel and mash up the ripe papaya in a glass or porcelain bowl. Apply the mashed pulp to your clean face, avoiding the eye area. Let it set for one to three minutes, or less if it tingles too much. Rinse off with warm water and apply a layer of fresh yogurt. Let set until yogurt dries, then rinse off with warm water and apply moisturizer. This is effective when mixed up immediately prior to applying.

Pineapple Enzyme Mask

½ cup of fresh (not canned) ripe pineapple
¼ cup of plain yogurt

Puree the pineapple in a blender and apply the juicy pulp to your clean skin, avoiding the eye area. Let set for about three minutes and rinse off. Apply a layer of yogurt to your face and let it set until the yogurt dries. Rinse off with warm water and apply moisturizer.

Papaya Pineapple Enzyme Mask

¼ cup of pureed fresh papaya
¼ cup of pureed fresh pineapple
¼ cup of plain yogurt

Mix the purees together and apply to your clean face, avoiding the eye area. Let set for about five minutes, then rinse off and apply moisturizer. Apply a layer of yogurt to your face and let set until it dries. Rinse off with warm water and apply moisturizer again.

Buttermilk Mask

This also acts as a mild exfoliator.

2 or 3 tablespoons of buttermilk

Apply a generous layer of buttermilk to clean skin. Let set until almost dry, then rinse off with warm water and apply toner and moisturizer.

Yogurt Mask

This is soothing as a mask and skin conditioner.

1 tablespoon of regular plain yogurt

Smooth a tablespoon of yogurt onto your clean face. Let the yogurt dry and rinse off with warm water. Apply moisturizer.

Clay Mask

**This is good for normal and oily skin;
it "deep" cleans and tightens.**

2 tablespoons of powdered kaolin

Buy powdered kaolin (clay) from your beauty supply or health store. One product I use is Magick Baby Powder, which is 100 percent kaolin. Mix 2 tablespoons of clay with warm water and apply it evenly to your face, avoiding the eye area. Let it dry thoroughly and then remove with a warm, wet washcloth. Be sure to remove all traces of the clay. Apply toner and moisturizer.

Milk of Magnesia Mask

**This is an excellent choice for oily skin.
The liquid magnesium absorbs oil.**

2 or 3 tablespoons of Milk of Magnesia

Just buy a bottle of plain Milk of Magnesia, shake it well to mix the product, and apply an even coat to your face. Let it absorb oil for about 15 to 20 minutes, then rinse away with warm water.

Yeast Mask

This is good for oily skin.

1 tablespoon of Brewer's yeast or a cake of fresh yeast

Look for brewer's yeast at your health store or supermarket. If the brewer's yeast is in powder form, mix about a tablespoon of it with enough water to make a paste. If the yeast is in cake form, break off about a tablespoon's worth and mix with water. Apply the paste to your face, avoiding the eye area. Let the mask harden, then remove with a washcloth saturated with warm water. Follow up with toner and moisturizer.

Honey Mask

This is good for dry skin and soothes irritations.

2 tablespoons of honey

Apply 2 tablespoons—an even layer—of honey to clean skin. Let it set for 15 minutes. Rinse off with warm water and follow up with toner and moisturizer.

Avocado Mask

This is good for dry skin.

½ ripe avocado

Mash avocado into a paste and apply to clean skin. Let it set for 20 minutes and rinse off with warm water. Follow up with toner and moisturizer.

Toners

These homemade toners work best when they are made fresh before each application. If this isn't convenient, you can make a few batches of it and store them in the refrigerator. They may last for about ten days, but let your nose and eyes be your guide. Making toners requires a blender. If you have a juicer that separates the pulp from the juice, it makes things a lot easier.

Grapefruit and Lemon Toner

This is good for oily skin.

Peel of 1 fresh lemon
Peel of 1 fresh grapefruit
2 cups of bottled or distilled water
1 tablespoon of witch hazel

Combine all of the ingredients except the witch hazel in a pan and bring to a slow boil. Cook until the peelings have softened. Cool and strain the mixture. Add witch hazel. Using a cotton pad, apply as a toner, then store the rest in the refrigerator.

Cucumber and Lemon Toner

This is good for normal to oily skin.

1 fresh cucumber
Juice of 1 fresh lemon
¼ cup of bottled or distilled water

Chop up the cucumber in large pieces and puree in a blender. Strain and add the lemon juice and water. Apply the toner to your skin with a cotton pad after cleansing and before moisturizing. Store in the refrigerator.

Fade Creams

If you'd like to try an alternative to commercial fade creams, try this.

Lemon Papaya Drops

Mix one drop of fresh papaya juice with one drop of fresh lemon juice. Dab on the dark spot every morning and evening. The papaya enzyme helps exfoliate the hyperpigmented spot and the lemon juice is a natural bleaching agent.

Pimple Treatment

Put one drop of lavender essential oil onto a piece of moistened cotton. Dab onto the blemish each day until it heals.

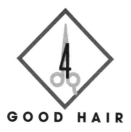

GOOD HAIR

While promoting my book *Good Hair*, I was interviewed by a reporter for the *Boston Herald* for a story about bad-hair days, specifically bad-weather days that required some sort of head covering. It took a little explaining because for some black women, the terms "bad hair" and "bad-hair day" are synonymous.

This chapter is meant to be informative, but I can't possibly put a book's worth of hair information into one chapter. Therefore, if you'd like more in-depth information about hair, read my previous books, *Good Hair: For Colored Girls Who've Considered Weaves When the Chemicals Became Too Ruff* and *Plaited Glory: For Colored Girls Who've Considered Braids, Locks, and Twists.*

Help Me, I've Stumbled and My Hair Won't Grow . . .

If you are diligent about the way you handle your hair, minimize or avoid the use of heated appliances, and avoid chemically overprocessing, you will prevent 95 percent of hair loss due to breakage. This sounds easy, but many women have *mindsets* and *arguments* that defeat their program. I'm not saying there is only one way to manage your hair. I *am* saying that physical manipulation, regular use of heated styling methods, and chemical overprocessing are the three major reasons for hair grief and that *your will to overcome* these stumbling blocks has much to do with your success rate.

Afrocentric Styles

Braids, locks, twists, and all their variations are great alternatives to straightening your hair or giving your chemically straightened hair a short respite from heated styling methods. I've included a sampling of styles here, but I've gone into great detail about the basics of maintaining these styles, as well as the lowdown on everything from choosing salons to tips for parents with style-hungry daughters, in *Plaited Glory: For Colored Girls Who've Considered Braids, Locks, and Twists.*

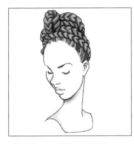

Goddess braids. Usually done with lin (wool fiber) extensions to pump up the volume. If you need a conservative look, go for a less intricate pattern. Lasts up to two weeks.

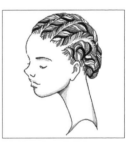

Flat twists or rolls. Hair is parted, twisted, and rolled into patterns. Can be as elaborate or as simple as you like.

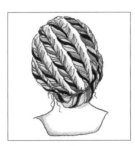

Flat twists, back view. This is another look that can go to the office. Lasts up to two weeks.

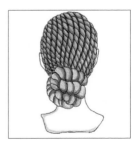

More flat twists. Think of these as two-strand cornrows. These can be done with or without lin extensions. They'll last for two weeks.

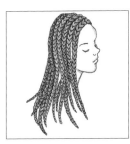

Individual Senegalese braids. The ends are tapered to give the look of real hair. Synthetic extensions will help these last for two or three months.

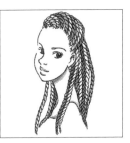

Individual two-strand Senegalese twists. These are done using synthetic hair extensions or lin. Lasts for three months.

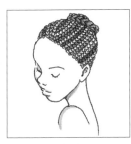

Cornrows. The classic standby. If you use extensions, they can last for two months. Without them, they'll last about two weeks.

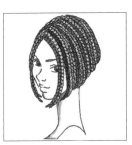

Bobbed individuals. The curved shape can be achieved by a braiding method called stitching, which creates tension in the ends of the braids and curves them. Synthetic extensions are often burned and softened in hot water. The ends can also be bumped with a curling iron.

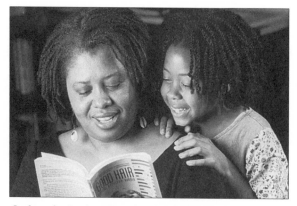

Locks and twists leave time for other mother-daughter activities.

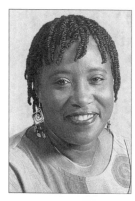 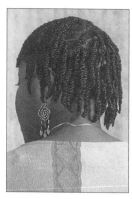

Glorries Daniels is styling two-strand twists that frame her face in a chic little bob. This style fits in perfectly with her career in the health-care industry.

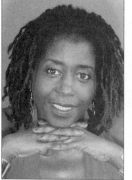 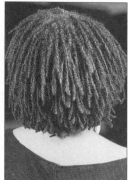

Queen Raziya—a master locktician with the locks to back it up.

Good hair means never having to worry about the back view.

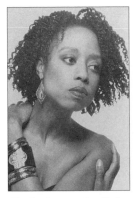

The "corkscrew crimp." A style created by twisting up damp hair, leaving it to dry, and then unfurling it.

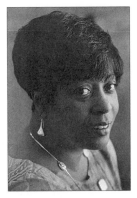

Mary Blanding is living proof that the right haircut makes all the difference. Her chemically relaxed bob is flattering and easy to maintain.

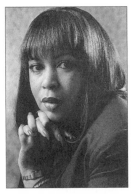

This is the result of a good relaxer, flat-ironing, cellophane for gloss, and wrapsetting at night. Learn how to work a perm so you can have hair like Dierdre's. Kudos to Rhonda, her beautician.

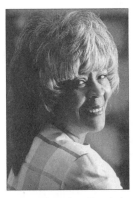

Yvonne keeps her silver hair lush and full by using a wrap set at night. Her beautician presses her hair and uses products that enhance its silvery white color.

DON'T HATE ME BECAUSE I WANT TO BE BEAUTIFUL

Somehow, in "Black Mythology," the idea of wearing makeup became mixed up with images of loose women, women who have rejected their racial identity, women who don't believe in God, and all sorts of other nonsense.

Well, I use makeup and I am neither loose nor racially conflicted. Some people say that only women who were raised by a mother who passed on makeup tips in utero or had five sisters who exchanged makeover tips every night instinctively know what the deal is when it comes to cosmetic enhancement. That's just hogwash. The true beauty mavens are the ones who were deprived of the woman's prerogative of wearing makeup. Women like me. Women who'd been denied for so long that it became an obsession. At one point I craved any exposure to beauty secrets that I could get.

My mother, who has been blessed with great, evenly pigmented skin, only wore lipstick. *Red* lipstick. None of those trendy frosts for her. In her day, folks were sensitive and conservative about attention-grabbing color on the face. A classic red was fine, but not too many respectable brown women walked around with brilliantly frosted or bright orange lips. My mother was fond of saying that she didn't want her lips entering a room before she did. She would take a tiny pink lipstick brush, fill it with color from the lipstick tube, and outline her lips. Then she'd fill them in with color and blot them with a tissue. Maybe she'd open a compact and wave the puff around her nose; she was always self-conscious about her makeup being too visible. That was her daily maquillage. (Not even eyebrow plucking, because she didn't believe in that.)

"I've just never gone in for the way these women tweeze all their

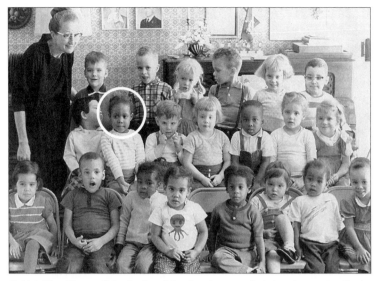

Robin's Nest Nursery School, where I developed my own fruit-based cosmetics. I'm in the second row biting my lips so they'll be red for the picture.

eyebrows away into these little arches and then they have to draw them back in," she'd say.

If my father happened to be listening, he'd always chime in with an "Amen."

I could see that lipstick was all I was going to get to work with in this house, so I started early.

My very first lipstick was a plastic bullet stolen from my brother's Lone Ranger gun and holster set. By the time I was five years old, me and the other girls would stain our lips and cheeks with the juice of wild cherries that we'd discovered in the nursery school play yard. Any traces of the cherry stain had to be removed by the time my mother came to pick me up, but until that time came, I was beautiful.

My mother didn't wear anything other than her lipstick and a dab of powder, but she had an Avon cosmetics lady who would give her samples of perfume and other cosmetics, mostly lipstick. I remember those samples quite fondly, because they were miniature lipsticks in white plastic cases, just the right size for a child. The Avon samples had the most appealing fragrance, a flowery, grown-up smell. Now, I knew better than to think I was going to be able to wear the stuff in public, but I craved the little cases and would beg for them after the lipstick sample was used up. This only happened if the samples were red shades because my mother wouldn't wear anything else. Still, I begged, but my parents were wary of a child having access to any sort of face paint and would not give up the goods. Luckily for me, there were other little girls whose mothers patronized the Avon lady and they passed on the samples for them to play with. They were sometimes willing to give me an empty case or two.

One day, my father spied me with a contraband lipstick case and came down on me like he was making a vice bust.

"And what do you think you're going to do with *this*?"

"Christina gave it to me, Daddy. I'm just *playing* with it." I was using my best wheedling here. "Please, *please*, can I keep it?"

The Inspector examined the little lipstick and discovered a dab of cosmetic in the bottom of the case. He had the evidence—would he come down on me? I decided to go for a three-tier defense.

"Aw, Daddy, it's just a little bit." I opened with the facts. Just lay them out, say it plain.

"I won't take it to school." Great declarative here—it showed a respect for authority and commitment.

"Please, can I keep it?" The close was simple and reinforced my goal of possession.

He reached a verdict in no time.

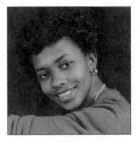

My naturally beautiful mother, who is blessed with the Blanding skin. She never wore anything more than lipstick and a dab of powder.

"So you can dig it out and spread it on your lips? You certainly may not!"

I guess he had visions of his six-year-old daughter entertaining ten-year-old boys with her frosted pink lips. I hadn't even thought that far ahead—I would have been happy just to keep the empty lipstick case. Foiled again.

I was also extremely fond of compacts. They were a perfect companion to lipstick, and I would imitate my mother snapping open hers and painting her lips. I was on the lookout for anything resem-